Advanced Soapmaking:
59 Recipes Of Soap Bars And Liquid Soaps For Regular Use And For Healing

Table of content

Book 1

Homesteading Soapmaking

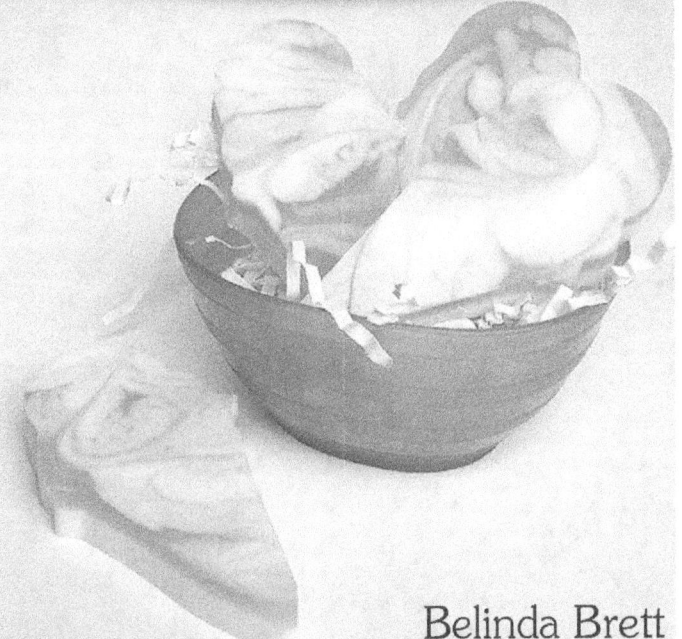

Belinda Brett

29 Recipes Of Liquid Soap And Soap Bars To Keep You Away From Mass Producing

Homesteading Soapmaking
29 Recipes Of Liquid Soap And Soap Bars To Keep You Away From Mass Producing

Introduction

When it comes to the world of soaps, it's easy to get confused. There are so many different soaps available on the market, and many of them say that the others are harmful in some way. But, when you keep hearing that the other soaps are bad, it can be hard to know when you are making the right option.

You do your best. You look around for a variety of different soaps, and you do what you can to make it work. However, the more you try to find the right soap for you, the more you hear that all the soaps are bad.

There are chemicals, there are harmful ingredients, there are all kinds of things you should never put on your skin. When it comes to the world of cleaners and soaps, you can easily feel like you are trapped in the same old cycle and never really doing your body and favors.

If only there was a way for you to make your own soaps. If only there was a way for you to know what was going into your soaps and what you are putting on your body. If only there was a way to know how to make your own soap the safe and easy way.

Now, there is.

With this book, you are going to learn everything you need to know to make your own soaps. You will learn how to use safe ingredients that are right for you, you will learn how to assemble these ingredients in a safe way, and you are going to learn how to blend rich scents that will make you feel like royalty every time you wash.

With these soaps, there are so many things you can do that you will fall in love with, and you will never want to go back to the conventional soaps again. Soon, you will see how expensive buying soap can be, and you will wonder what you have been putting on your skin all this time.

This book is going to change the way you view your soaps, and how you take care of your skin. You are going to fall in love with the results, and you are going to realize just how well you can pamper your skin. There are so many things you can do to keep your skin bright and healthy.

Let this book show you how you can treat your skin the right way, and give yourself a pampering spa treatment every time you step in the tub.

You know you want to, and you know that it's possible, so why not dive in with both feet?

Love the skin you're in.

Chapter 1 – The Liquid Soaps

World's Best Body Wash

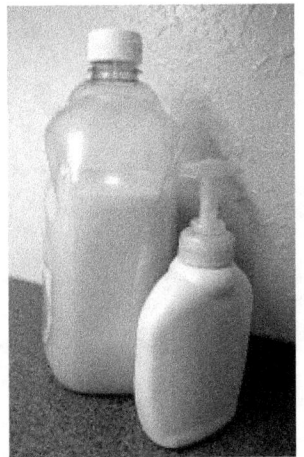

What you will need:

10 drops rose oil

8 drops rosewood oil

½ cup fractionated coconut oil

¼ cup witch hazel

2 tablespoons rubbing alcohol

1 cup shea butter

Directions:

Place water in your double boiler and turn the boiler on. Melt the shea butter completely, then add all remaining ingredients except for the essential oils. Continue to stir until the mix is completely blended.

Add in the essential oils.

Remove the mix from heat and allow to cool on your counter. Use a whisk or hand mixer to whisk the soap as it slows – about once every half hour. Pour the liquid soap into a pump and store by your kitchen or bathroom sinks. Use as needed.

Sudsy Hand Soap

What you will need:

10 drops sunflower oil

6 drops geranium oil

½ cup fractionated coconut oil

¼ cup witch hazel

2 tablespoons rubbing alcohol

1 cup shea butter

Directions:

Place water in your double boiler and turn the boiler on. Melt the shea butter completely, then add all remaining ingredients except for the essential oils. Continue to stir until the mix is completely blended.

Add in the essential oils.

Remove the mix from heat and allow to cool on your counter. Use a whisk or hand mixer to whisk the soap as it slows – about once every half hour. Pour the liquid soap into a pump and store by your kitchen or bathroom sinks. Use as needed.

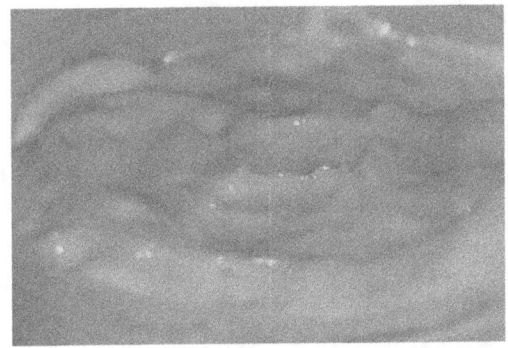

Wonder Wash
What you will need:

12 drops bergamot oil

10 drops vetiver oil

½ cup fractionated coconut oil

¼ cup witch hazel

2 tablespoons rubbing alcohol

1 cup shea butter

Directions:

Place water in your double boiler and turn the boiler on. Melt the shea butter completely, then add all remaining ingredients except for the essential oils. Continue to stir until the mix is completely blended.

Add in the essential oils.

Remove the mix from heat and allow to cool on your counter. Use a whisk or hand mixer to whisk the soap as it slows – about once every half hour. Pour the liquid soap into a pump and store by your kitchen or bathroom sinks. Use as needed.

All About Those Bubbles

What you will need:

10 drops bubblegum scented oil

8 drops rose oil

½ cup fractionated coconut oil

¼ cup witch hazel

2 tablespoons rubbing alcohol

1 cup shea butter

Directions:

Place water in your double boiler and turn the boiler on. Melt the shea butter completely, then add all remaining ingredients except for the essential oils. Continue to stir until the mix is completely blended.

Add in the essential oils.

Remove the mix from heat and allow to cool on your counter. Use a whisk or hand mixer to whisk the soap as it slows – about once every half hour. Pour the liquid soap into a pump and store by your kitchen or bathroom sinks. Use as needed.

Happy Days Hand Wash

What you will need:

12 drops clary sage oil

8 drops frankincense oil

½ cup fractionated coconut oil

¼ cup witch hazel

2 tablespoons rubbing alcohol

1 cup shea butter

Directions:

Place water in your double boiler and turn the boiler on. Melt the shea butter completely, then add all remaining ingredients except for the essential oils. Continue to stir until the mix is completely blended.

Add in the essential oils.

Remove the mix from heat and allow to cool on your counter. Use a whisk or hand mixer to whisk the soap as it slows – about once every half hour. Pour the liquid soap into a pump and store by your kitchen or bathroom sinks. Use as needed.

Hello Sunshine

What you will need:

12 drops lemongrass oil

8 drops lemon

½ cup fractionated coconut oil

¼ cup witch hazel

2 tablespoons rubbing alcohol

1 cup shea butter

Directions:

Place water in your double boiler and turn the boiler on. Melt the shea butter completely, then add all remaining ingredients except for the essential oils. Continue to stir until the mix is completely blended.

Add in the essential oils.

Remove the mix from heat and allow to cool on your counter. Use a whisk or hand mixer to whisk the soap as it slows – about once every half hour. Pour the liquid soap into a pump and store by your kitchen or bathroom sinks. Use as needed.

Bath Time

What you will need:

18 drops myrrh oil

12 drops lavender oil

½ cup fractionated coconut oil

¼ cup witch hazel

2 tablespoons rubbing alcohol

1 cup shea butter

Directions:

Place water in your double boiler and turn the boiler on. Melt the shea butter completely, then add all remaining ingredients except for the essential oils. Continue to stir until the mix is completely blended.

Add in the essential oils.

Remove the mix from heat and allow to cool on your counter. Use a whisk or hand mixer to whisk the soap as it slows – about once every half hour. Pour the liquid soap into a pump and store by your kitchen or bathroom sinks. Use as needed.

Heavenly Flowers

What you will need:

12 drops ylang ylang oil

8 drops neem oil

½ cup fractionated coconut oil

¼ cup witch hazel

2 tablespoons rubbing alcohol

1 cup shea butter

Directions:

Place water in your double boiler and turn the boiler on. Melt the shea butter completely, then add all remaining ingredients except for the essential oils. Continue to stir until the mix is completely blended.

Add in the essential oils.

Remove the mix from heat and allow to cool on your counter. Use a whisk or hand mixer to whisk the soap as it slows – about once every half hour. Pour the liquid soap into a pump and store by your kitchen or bathroom sinks. Use as needed.

Beautiful Day

What you will need:

12 drops basil oil

12 drops lavender oil

½ cup fractionated coconut oil

¼ cup witch hazel

2 tablespoons rubbing alcohol

1 cup shea butter

Directions:

Place water in your double boiler and turn the boiler on. Melt the shea butter completely, then add all remaining ingredients except for the essential oils. Continue to stir until the mix is completely blended.

Add in the essential oils.

Remove the mix from heat and allow to cool on your counter. Use a whisk or hand mixer to whisk the soap as it slows – about once every half hour. Pour the liquid soap into a pump and store by your kitchen or bathroom sinks. Use as needed.

Bath Bash

What you will need:

12 drops ginger oil

13 drops clary sage oil

½ cup fractionated coconut oil

¼ cup witch hazel

2 tablespoons rubbing alcohol

1 cup shea butter

Directions:

Place water in your double boiler and turn the boiler on. Melt the shea butter completely, then add all remaining ingredients except for the essential oils. Continue to stir until the mix is completely blended.

Add in the essential oils.

Remove the mix from heat and allow to cool on your counter. Use a whisk or hand mixer to whisk the soap as it slows – about once every half hour. Pour the liquid soap into a pump and store by your kitchen or bathroom sinks. Use as needed.

Very Berry Bubble Bath

What you will need:

12 drops vetiver oil

9 drops tarragon oil

½ cup fractionated coconut oil

¼ cup witch hazel

2 tablespoons rubbing alcohol

1 cup shea butter

Directions:

Place water in your double boiler and turn the boiler on. Melt the shea butter completely, then add all remaining ingredients except for the essential oils. Continue to stir until the mix is completely blended.

Add in the essential oils.

Remove the mix from heat and allow to cool on your counter. Use a whisk or hand mixer to whisk the soap as it slows – about once every half hour. Pour the liquid soap into a pump and store by your kitchen or bathroom sinks. Use as needed.

Clean Thing

What you will need:

12 drops cinnamon oil

10 drops cayenne oil

½ cup fractionated coconut oil

¼ cup witch hazel

2 tablespoons rubbing alcohol

1 cup shea butter

Directions:

Place water in your double boiler and turn the boiler on. Melt the shea butter completely, then add all remaining ingredients except for the essential oils. Continue to stir until the mix is completely blended.

Add in the essential oils.

Remove the mix from heat and allow to cool on your counter. Use a whisk or hand mixer to whisk the soap as it slows – about once every half hour. Pour the liquid soap into a pump and store by your kitchen or bathroom sinks. Use as needed.

Suds 'N' Buds
What you will need:

15 drops marjoram oil

9 drops clove oil

½ cup fractionated coconut oil

¼ cup witch hazel

2 tablespoons rubbing alcohol

1 cup shea butter

Directions:

Place water in your double boiler and turn the boiler on. Melt the shea butter completely, then add all remaining ingredients except for the essential oils. Continue to stir until the mix is completely blended.

Add in the essential oils.

Remove the mix from heat and allow to cool on your counter. Use a whisk or hand mixer to whisk the soap as it slows – about once every half hour. Pour the liquid soap into a pump and store by your kitchen or bathroom sinks. Use as needed.

Dirt Be gone
What you will need:

12 drops rooibos oil

12 drops cedar oil

½ cup fractionated coconut oil

¼ cup witch hazel

2 tablespoons rubbing alcohol

1 cup shea butter

Directions:

Place water in your double boiler and turn the boiler on. Melt the shea butter completely, then add all remaining ingredients except for the essential oils. Continue to stir until the mix is completely blended.

Add in the essential oils.

Remove the mix from heat and allow to cool on your counter. Use a whisk or hand mixer to whisk the soap as it slows – about once every half hour. Pour the liquid soap into a pump and store by your kitchen or bathroom sinks. Use as needed.

Relaxation Station
What you will need:

11 drops lavender oil

11 drops myrrh oil

½ cup fractionated coconut oil

¼ cup witch hazel

2 tablespoons rubbing alcohol

1 cup shea butter

Directions:

Place water in your double boiler and turn the boiler on. Melt the shea butter completely, then add all remaining ingredients except for the essential oils. Continue to stir until the mix is completely blended.

Add in the essential oils.

Remove the mix from heat and allow to cool on your counter. Use a whisk or hand mixer to whisk the soap as it slows – about once every half hour. Pour the liquid soap into a pump and store by your kitchen or bathroom sinks. Use as needed.

Chapter 2 – The Bar Soaps

Build a Bar Soap

What you will need:

12 drops neem oil

3 drops cinnamon oil

1 bar unscented white bar soap

3 tablespoons coconut oil

2 tablespoons almond oil

Directions:

Cut the bar into much smaller pieces, or run it through your blender and break it into shreds.

Prepare your double boiler, then place the soap inside. Add the coconut oil and almond oil and stir.

Continue to stir as the soap melts completely and once it has, add in the essential oils.

Remove from heat and allow to cool slightly, then transfer the soap mix into the molds. Allow to sit undisturbed overnight, and remove from molds in the morning.

Store in a dry place.

Gentle enough to be used on all parts of the body, and you can use it as often as you prefer.

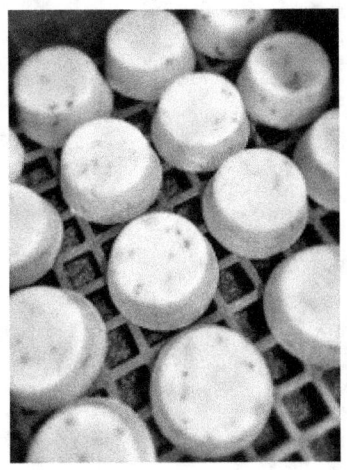

Basket Case

What you will need:

15 drops geranium oil

10 drops rose oil

1 bar unscented white bar soap

3 tablespoons coconut oil

2 tablespoons almond oil

Directions:

Cut the bar into much smaller pieces, or run it through your blender and break it into shreds.

Prepare your double boiler, then place the soap inside. Add the coconut oil and almond oil and stir.

Continue to stir as the soap melts completely and once it has, add in the essential oils.

Remove from heat and allow to cool slightly, then transfer the soap mix into the molds. Allow to sit undisturbed overnight, and remove from molds in the morning.

Store in a dry place.

Gentle enough to be used on all parts of the body, and you can use it as often as you prefer.

Bath and Body Bar

What you will need:

19 drops neroli oil

12 drops basil oil

1 bar unscented white bar soap

3 tablespoons coconut oil

2 tablespoons almond oil

Directions:

Cut the bar into much smaller pieces, or run it through your blender and break it into shreds.

Prepare your double boiler, then place the soap inside. Add the coconut oil and almond oil and stir.

Continue to stir as the soap melts completely and once it has, add in the essential oils.

Remove from heat and allow to cool slightly, then transfer the soap mix into the molds. Allow to sit undisturbed overnight, and remove from molds in the morning.

Store in a dry place.

Gentle enough to be used on all parts of the body, and you can use it as often as you prefer.

The High Bar
What you will need:

15 drops frankincense oil

12 drops myrrh oil

1 bar unscented white bar soap

3 tablespoons coconut oil

2 tablespoons almond oil

Directions:

Cut the bar into much smaller pieces, or run it through your blender and break it into shreds.

Prepare your double boiler, then place the soap inside. Add the coconut oil and almond oil and stir.

Continue to stir as the soap melts completely and once it has, add in the essential oils.

Remove from heat and allow to cool slightly, then transfer the soap mix into the molds. Allow to sit undisturbed overnight, and remove from molds in the morning.

Store in a dry place.

Gentle enough to be used on all parts of the body, and you can use it as often as you prefer.

Honey Bar

What you will need:

12 drops lavender oil

12 drops rose oil

1 tablespoon honey

1 bar unscented white bar soap

3 tablespoons coconut oil

2 tablespoons almond oil

Directions:

Cut the bar into much smaller pieces, or run it through your blender and break it into shreds.

Prepare your double boiler, then place the soap inside. Add the coconut oil and almond oil and stir.

Continue to stir as the soap melts completely and once it has, add in the essential oils.

Remove from heat and allow to cool slightly, then transfer the soap mix into the molds. Allow to sit undisturbed overnight, and remove from molds in the morning.

Store in a dry place.

Gentle enough to be used on all parts of the body, and you can use it as often as you prefer.

Bubble Bar

What you will need:

12 drops green apple scented oil

10 drops pine oil

1 bar unscented white bar soap

3 tablespoons coconut oil

2 tablespoons almond oil

Directions:

Cut the bar into much smaller pieces, or run it through your blender and break it into shreds.

Prepare your double boiler, then place the soap inside. Add the coconut oil and almond oil and stir.

Continue to stir as the soap melts completely and once it has, add in the essential oils.

Remove from heat and allow to cool slightly, then transfer the soap mix into the molds. Allow to sit undisturbed overnight, and remove from molds in the morning.

Store in a dry place.

Gentle enough to be used on all parts of the body, and you can use it as often as you prefer.

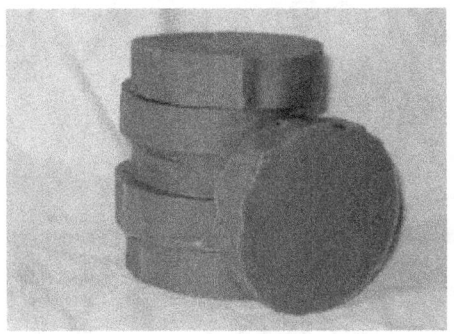

For the Bar

What you will need:

12 drops lemongrass oil

10 drops lemon oil

1 bar unscented white bar soap

3 tablespoons coconut oil

2 tablespoons almond oil

Directions:

Cut the bar into much smaller pieces, or run it through your blender and break it into shreds.

Prepare your double boiler, then place the soap inside. Add the coconut oil and almond oil and stir.

Continue to stir as the soap melts completely and once it has, add in the essential oils.

Remove from heat and allow to cool slightly, then transfer the soap mix into the molds. Allow to sit undisturbed overnight, and remove from molds in the morning.

Store in a dry place.

Gentle enough to be used on all parts of the body, and you can use it as often as you prefer.

King Bar

What you will need:

18 drops wintergreen oil

12 drops fir needle oil

1 bar unscented white bar soap

3 tablespoons coconut oil

2 tablespoons almond oil

Directions:

Cut the bar into much smaller pieces, or run it through your blender and break it into shreds.

Prepare your double boiler, then place the soap inside. Add the coconut oil and almond oil and stir.

Continue to stir as the soap melts completely and once it has, add in the essential oils.

Remove from heat and allow to cool slightly, then transfer the soap mix into the molds. Allow to sit undisturbed overnight, and remove from molds in the morning.

Store in a dry place.

Gentle enough to be used on all parts of the body, and you can use it as often as you prefer.

The Bar of Perfection
What you will need:

15 drops vetiver oil

12 drops ylang ylang oil

1 bar unscented white bar soap

3 tablespoons coconut oil

2 tablespoons almond oil

Directions:

Cut the bar into much smaller pieces, or run it through your blender and break it into shreds.

Prepare your double boiler, then place the soap inside. Add the coconut oil and almond oil and stir.

Continue to stir as the soap melts completely and once it has, add in the essential oils.

Remove from heat and allow to cool slightly, then transfer the soap mix into the molds. Allow to sit undisturbed overnight, and remove from molds in the morning.

Store in a dry place.

Gentle enough to be used on all parts of the body, and you can use it as often as you prefer.

Because Bar
What you will need:

12 drops grapefruit oil

10 drops lemon oil

12 drops orange oil

1 bar unscented white bar soap

3 tablespoons coconut oil

2 tablespoons almond oil

Directions:

Cut the bar into much smaller pieces, or run it through your blender and break it into shreds.

Prepare your double boiler, then place the soap inside. Add the coconut oil and almond oil and stir.

Continue to stir as the soap melts completely and once it has, add in the essential oils.

Remove from heat and allow to cool slightly, then transfer the soap mix into the molds. Allow to sit undisturbed overnight, and remove from molds in the morning.

Store in a dry place.

Gentle enough to be used on all parts of the body, and you can use it as often as you prefer.

Beauty Bar

What you will need:

12 drops neem oil

10 drops geranium oil

1 bar unscented white bar soap

3 tablespoons coconut oil

2 tablespoons almond oil

Directions:

Cut the bar into much smaller pieces, or run it through your blender and break it into shreds.

Prepare your double boiler, then place the soap inside. Add the coconut oil and almond oil and stir.

Continue to stir as the soap melts completely and once it has, add in the essential oils.

Remove from heat and allow to cool slightly, then transfer the soap mix into the molds. Allow to sit undisturbed overnight, and remove from molds in the morning.

Store in a dry place.

Gentle enough to be used on all parts of the body, and you can use it as often as you prefer.

Bring Back the Bar

What you will need:

15 drops bergamot oil

12 drops watermelon scented oil

1 bar unscented white bar soap

3 tablespoons coconut oil

2 tablespoons almond oil

Directions:

Cut the bar into much smaller pieces, or run it through your blender and break it into shreds.

Prepare your double boiler, then place the soap inside. Add the coconut oil and almond oil and stir.

Continue to stir as the soap melts completely and once it has, add in the essential oils.

Remove from heat and allow to cool slightly, then transfer the soap mix into the molds. Allow to sit undisturbed overnight, and remove from molds in the morning.

Store in a dry place.

Gentle enough to be used on all parts of the body, and you can use it as often as you prefer.

The Jar Bar

What you will need:

12 drops cinnamon oil

12 drops vanilla oil

1 bar unscented white bar soap

3 tablespoons coconut oil

2 tablespoons almond oil

Directions:

Cut the bar into much smaller pieces, or run it through your blender and break it into shreds.

Prepare your double boiler, then place the soap inside. Add the coconut oil and almond oil and stir.

Continue to stir as the soap melts completely and once it has, add in the essential oils.

Remove from heat and allow to cool slightly, then transfer the soap mix into the molds. Allow to sit undisturbed overnight, and remove from molds in the morning.

Store in a dry place.

Gentle enough to be used on all parts of the body, and you can use it as often as you prefer.

True Bar
What you will need:

12 drops orange oil

10 drops blood orange oil

1 bar unscented white bar soap

3 tablespoons coconut oil

2 tablespoons almond oil

Directions:

Cut the bar into much smaller pieces, or run it through your blender and break it into shreds.

Prepare your double boiler, then place the soap inside. Add the coconut oil and almond oil and stir.

Continue to stir as the soap melts completely and once it has, add in the essential oils.

Remove from heat and allow to cool slightly, then transfer the soap mix into the molds. Allow to sit undisturbed overnight, and remove from molds in the morning.

Store in a dry place.

Gentle enough to be used on all parts of the body, and you can use it as often as you prefer.

The Daily Bar

What you will need:

14 drops ylang ylang oil

9 drops juniper berry oil

1 bar unscented white bar soap

3 tablespoons coconut oil

2 tablespoons almond oil

Directions:

Cut the bar into much smaller pieces, or run it through your blender and break it into shreds.

Prepare your double boiler, then place the soap inside. Add the coconut oil and almond oil and stir.

Continue to stir as the soap melts completely and once it has, add in the essential oils.

Remove from heat and allow to cool slightly, then transfer the soap mix into the molds. Allow to sit undisturbed overnight, and remove from molds in the morning.

Store in a dry place.

Gentle enough to be used on all parts of the body, and you can use it as often as you prefer.

Conclusion

There you have it, everything you need to know to make your own soap at home, no matter what kind of soap you wish to make. There are all kinds of different soaps you can make, and when you are using your own scents, you can make it entirely your own.

I hope this book inspires you to create a variety of your own soaps, and that you take what you have learned here and apply them to the soaps you wish to create. There's no end to the ways you can show off your style, and when it comes to the world of homemade soaps, you can do that very thing.

This book is the secret you have been looking for, making it possible for anyone to make any kind of soap they want, regardless of their budget or whether they have small children or pets around the hobby.

You deserve to be pampered and you deserve to love the time you spend in the tub, and when you are using these soaps, you are going to get that very thing.

I hope this book opens the door to a whole new level of pampering for you, and that you make each and every one of these soaps. Use the recipes as they are, and mix and match to create your own unique scents. There are so many different ways you can show off your signature scent.

You are going to fall in love with these recipes, and I know they are going to change the way you pamper yourself in the evening. You are going to love the results, and you are going to find that from the very first time you wash, your skin will thank you.

Dive into the world of clean living with both feet, and you are going to find that your bath may be the very best part of your day.

HEALING SOAP RECIPES

30 HOMEMADE SOAPS THAT CURE SKIN PROBLEMS

RONDA WILLSON

Healing Soap Recipes
30 Homemade Soaps That Cure Skin Problems

Introduction

You know germs are everywhere, and you know in order to stay healthy, you are going to have to keep clean. But, it seems that there is always something going on with your skin that drives you insane – whether you are dealing with burns, scraps, dry skin, irritation, or rashes.

The soaps on the market can be harsh on these conditions, making it harder for you to heal. But, you can't give up on using these soaps, or you are going to risk infections, illness, and a host of other problems.

So what are you going to do?

Clearly, the answer is to make your own soap.

But, you wonder, how are you going to do this – isn't soap difficult to make? Aren't there all kinds of harmful ingredients involved? Is there any way you can do it and not risk exposure to harmful chemicals?

If you have ever had any of these concerns, you have come to the right place. This book is going to show you everything you need to know to make your own soaps, regardless of what your skin irritation is.

Discover a host of different recipes, and create the soap that is going to get you back on track, and fall in love with being clean.

Chapter 1 – Healing Soaps for Dry Skin

Whether it is the cold of winter or the heat of summer, it seems that you can't get away from the dry skin that plagues you. Thankfully, you do have relief in sight, and with these soaps, you are going to get that moisture your dry skin so desperately needs.

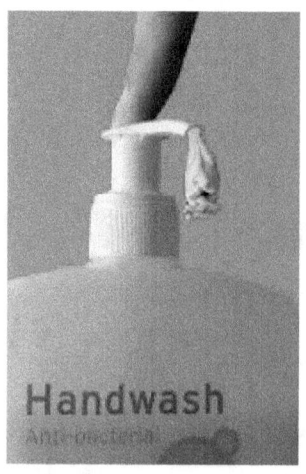

Moisture Extreme
What you will need:

12 drops chamomile essential oil

12 drops myrrh essential oil

1 tablespoon honey

1 cup unscented castile soap

2 tablespoons shea butter

1 tablespoon glycerin

¼ cup distilled water

Directions:

Using either a double boiler or a homemade double boiler, melt the shea butter until it is completely smooth. Add in the remaining ingredients (except for the essential oils) one at a time, mixing them in thoroughly (you don't want there to be any lumps in the mix at all.)

After you have thoroughly blended the ingredients, add the essential oils in next, and also stir them in until the mix is completely smooth. Remove from heat and allow to cool slightly, stirring the entire time.

Once the soap has cooled enough to touch, transfer from your double boiler to a soap dispenser, and use frequently on any dry skin you have.

Soothing Oasis

What you will need:

10 drops sunflower essential oil

10 drops sandalwood oil

1 tablespoon honey

1 cup unscented castile soap

2 tablespoons shea butter

1 tablespoon glycerin

¼ cup distilled water

Directions:

Using either a double boiler or a homemade double boiler, melt the shea butter until it is completely smooth. Add in the remaining ingredients (except for the essential oils) one at a time, mixing them in thoroughly (you don't want there to be any lumps in the mix at all.)

After you have thoroughly blended the ingredients, add the essential oils in next, and also stir them in until the mix is completely smooth. Remove from heat and allow to cool slightly, stirring the entire time.

Once the soap has cooled enough to touch, transfer from your double boiler to a soap dispenser, and use frequently on any dry skin you have.

Skip to My Loo
What you will need:

10 drops juniper berry essential oil

12 drops clove oil

1 tablespoon honey

1 cup unscented castile soap

2 tablespoons shea butter

1 tablespoon glycerin

¼ cup distilled water

Directions:

Using either a double boiler or a homemade double boiler, melt the shea butter until it is completely smooth. Add in the remaining ingredients (except for the essential oils) one at a time, mixing them in thoroughly (you don't want there to be any lumps in the mix at all.)

After you have thoroughly blended the ingredients, add the essential oils in next, and also stir them in until the mix is completely smooth. Remove from heat and allow to cool slightly, stirring the entire time.

Once the soap has cooled enough to touch, transfer from your double boiler to a soap dispenser, and use frequently on any dry skin you have.

Silken Fingers
What you will need:

18 drops vanilla essential oil

12 drops lavender essential oil

1 tablespoon honey

1 cup unscented castile soap

2 tablespoons shea butter

1 tablespoon glycerin

¼ cup distilled water

Directions:

Using either a double boiler or a homemade double boiler, melt the shea butter until it is completely smooth. Add in the remaining ingredients (except for the essential oils) one at a time, mixing them in thoroughly (you don't want there to be any lumps in the mix at all.)

After you have thoroughly blended the ingredients, add the essential oils in next, and also stir them in until the mix is completely smooth. Remove from heat and allow to cool slightly, stirring the entire time.

Once the soap has cooled enough to touch, transfer from your double boiler to a soap dispenser, and use frequently on any dry skin you have.

Happy Hands
What you will need:

10 drops rose essential oil

10 drops myrrh essential oil

1 tablespoon honey

1 cup unscented castile soap

2 tablespoons shea butter

1 tablespoon glycerin

¼ cup distilled water

Directions:

Using either a double boiler or a homemade double boiler, melt the shea butter until it is completely smooth. Add in the remaining ingredients (except for the essential oils) one at a time, mixing them in thoroughly (you don't want there to be any lumps in the mix at all.)

After you have thoroughly blended the ingredients, add the essential oils in next, and also stir them in until the mix is completely smooth. Remove from heat and allow to cool slightly, stirring the entire time.

Once the soap has cooled enough to touch, transfer from your double boiler to a soap dispenser, and use frequently on any dry skin you have.

Better than Oil

What you will need:

12 drops grapefruit oil

10 drops sunflower essential oil

1 tablespoon honey

1 cup unscented castile soap

2 tablespoons shea butter

1 tablespoon glycerin

¼ cup distilled water

Directions:

Using either a double boiler or a homemade double boiler, melt the shea butter until it is completely smooth. Add in the remaining ingredients (except for the essential oils) one at a time, mixing them in thoroughly (you don't want there to be any lumps in the mix at all.)

After you have thoroughly blended the ingredients, add the essential oils in next, and also stir them in until the mix is completely smooth. Remove from heat and allow to cool slightly, stirring the entire time.

Once the soap has cooled enough to touch, transfer from your double boiler to a soap dispenser, and use frequently on any dry skin you have.

Chapter 2 – Healing Soaps for Cuts, Scrapes, and Scratches

Whether it's you or your kids, there always seems to be someone with a scrape or a scratch in the house. With this soap, you can rest assured that those little injuries will heal quickly, ensuring you get a speedy recovery.

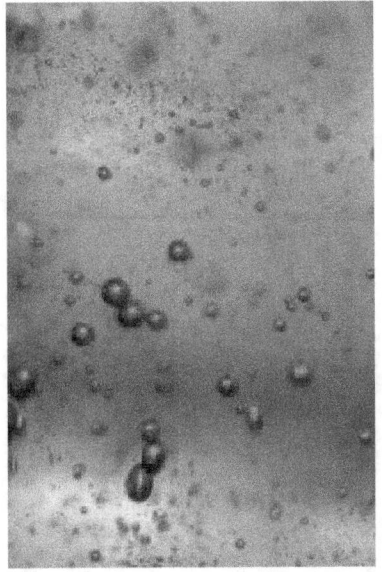

Clean Freak
What you will need:

12 drops cinnamon oil

6 drops orange oil

¼ teaspoon tea tree oil

1 cup unscented castile soap

1 tablespoon glycerin

¼ cup distilled water

Directions:

Using either a double boiler or a homemade double boiler, combine all ingredients (except for the essential oils) one at a time, mixing them together thoroughly.

After you have thoroughly blended the ingredients, add the essential oils in next, and also stir them in until the mix is completely smooth. Remove from heat and allow to cool slightly, stirring the entire time.

Once the soap has cooled enough to touch, transfer from your double boiler to a soap dispenser, and use frequently on any cuts or scrapes you have.

Kiss it Better
What you will need:

10 drops ylang ylang oil

12 drops cedar oil

¼ teaspoon tea tree oil

1 cup unscented castile soap

1 tablespoon glycerin

¼ cup distilled water

Directions:

Using either a double boiler or a homemade double boiler, combine all ingredients (except for the essential oils) one at a time, mixing them together thoroughly.

After you have thoroughly blended the ingredients, add the essential oils in next, and also stir them in until the mix is completely smooth. Remove from heat and allow to cool slightly, stirring the entire time.

Once the soap has cooled enough to touch, transfer from your double boiler to a soap dispenser, and use frequently on any cuts or scrapes you have.

Speed Healer
What you will need:

10 drops sage oil

10 drops clary sage oil

¼ teaspoon tea tree oil

1 cup unscented castile soap

1 tablespoon glycerin

¼ cup distilled water

Directions:

Using either a double boiler or a homemade double boiler, combine all ingredients (except for the essential oils) one at a time, mixing them together thoroughly.

After you have thoroughly blended the ingredients, add the essential oils in next, and also stir them in until the mix is completely smooth. Remove from heat and allow to cool slightly, stirring the entire time.

Once the soap has cooled enough to touch, transfer from your double boiler to a soap dispenser, and use frequently on any cuts or scrapes you have.

The Perfect Touch
What you will need:

12 drops lavender oil

10 drops sandalwood oil

¼ teaspoon tea tree oil

1 cup unscented castile soap

1 tablespoon glycerin

¼ cup distilled water

Directions:

Using either a double boiler or a homemade double boiler, combine all ingredients (except for the essential oils) one at a time, mixing them together thoroughly.

After you have thoroughly blended the ingredients, add the essential oils in next, and also stir them in until the mix is completely smooth. Remove from heat and allow to cool slightly, stirring the entire time.

Once the soap has cooled enough to touch, transfer from your double boiler to a soap dispenser, and use frequently on any cuts or scrapes you have.

Mother's Choice
What you will need:

10 drops lemongrass oil

10 drops lemon oil

¼ teaspoon tea tree oil

1 cup unscented castile soap

1 tablespoon glycerin

¼ cup distilled water

Directions:

Using either a double boiler or a homemade double boiler, combine all ingredients (except for the essential oils) one at a time, mixing them together thoroughly.

After you have thoroughly blended the ingredients, add the essential oils in next, and also stir them in until the mix is completely smooth. Remove from heat and allow to cool slightly, stirring the entire time.

Once the soap has cooled enough to touch, transfer from your double boiler to a soap dispenser, and use frequently on any cuts or scrapes you have.

Double Trouble

What you will need:

10 drops lemon oil

8 drops orange oil

¼ teaspoon tea tree oil

1 cup unscented castile soap

1 tablespoon glycerin

¼ cup distilled water

Directions:

Using either a double boiler or a homemade double boiler, combine all ingredients (except for the essential oils) one at a time, mixing them together thoroughly.

After you have thoroughly blended the ingredients, add the essential oils in next, and also stir them in until the mix is completely smooth. Remove from heat and allow to cool slightly, stirring the entire time.

Once the soap has cooled enough to touch, transfer from your double boiler to a soap dispenser, and use frequently on any cuts or scrapes you have.

Chapter 3 – Healing Soaps for Burns

No matter how careful you are in the kitchen, you are always risking being burned. When it does happen, you want relief, and you want it fast – and that's where these soaps come in. Wash your hands with these, and feel instant, soothing relief that will get you back in the game in no time.

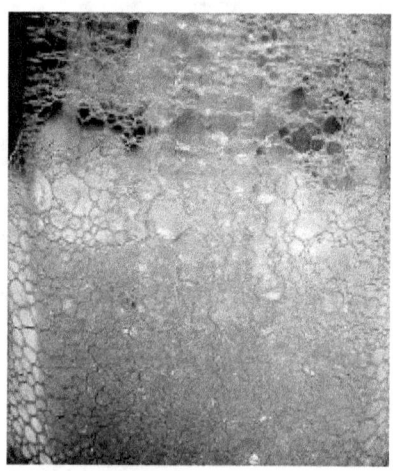

Baker's Best Friend
What you will need:

12 drops frankincense oil

10 drops jasmine oil

¼ cup aloe

1 tablespoon beeswax

1 cup unscented castile soap

1 tablespoon glycerin

¼ cup distilled water

Directions:

Using either a double boiler or a homemade double boiler, melt the beeswax until it is completely smooth. Add in the remaining ingredients (except for the essential oils) one at a time, mixing them in thoroughly (you don't want there to be any lumps in the mix at all.)

After you have thoroughly blended the ingredients, add the essential oils in next, and also stir them in until the mix is completely smooth. Remove from heat and allow to cool slightly, stirring the entire time.

Once the soap has cooled enough to touch, transfer from your double boiler to a soap dispenser, and use frequently on any burns you have.

The Fire Extinguisher
What you will need:

10 drops lavender oil

10 drops bergamot oil

¼ cup aloe

1 tablespoon beeswax

1 cup unscented castile soap

1 tablespoon glycerin

¼ cup distilled water

Directions:

Using either a double boiler or a homemade double boiler, melt the beeswax until it is completely smooth. Add in the remaining ingredients (except for the essential oils) one at a time, mixing them in thoroughly (you don't want there to be any lumps in the mix at all.)

After you have thoroughly blended the ingredients, add the essential oils in next, and also stir them in until the mix is completely smooth. Remove from heat and allow to cool slightly, stirring the entire time.

Once the soap has cooled enough to touch, transfer from your double boiler to a soap dispenser, and use frequently on any burns you have.

Burn Be Gone

What you will need:

12 drops tea tree oil

10 drops neem oil

¼ cup aloe

1 tablespoon beeswax

1 cup unscented castile soap

1 tablespoon glycerin

¼ cup distilled water

Directions:

Using either a double boiler or a homemade double boiler, melt the beeswax until it is completely smooth. Add in the remaining ingredients (except for the essential oils) one at a time, mixing them in thoroughly (you don't want there to be any lumps in the mix at all.)

After you have thoroughly blended the ingredients, add the essential oils in next, and also stir them in until the mix is completely smooth. Remove from heat and allow to cool slightly, stirring the entire time.

Once the soap has cooled enough to touch, transfer from your double boiler to a soap dispenser, and use frequently on any burns you have.

Splash
What you will need:

12 drops vetiver oil

10 drops sandalwood oil

¼ cup aloe

1 tablespoon beeswax

1 cup unscented castile soap

1 tablespoon glycerin

¼ cup distilled water

Directions:

Using either a double boiler or a homemade double boiler, melt the beeswax until it is completely smooth. Add in the remaining ingredients (except for the essential oils) one at a time, mixing them in thoroughly (you don't want there to be any lumps in the mix at all.)

After you have thoroughly blended the ingredients, add the essential oils in next, and also stir them in until the mix is completely smooth. Remove from heat and allow to cool slightly, stirring the entire time.

Once the soap has cooled enough to touch, transfer from your double boiler to a soap dispenser, and use frequently on any burns you have.

Cooling Contact
What you will need:

12 drops peppermint oil

10 drops eucalyptus oil

¼ cup aloe

1 tablespoon beeswax

1 cup unscented castile soap

1 tablespoon glycerin

¼ cup distilled water

Directions:

Using either a double boiler or a homemade double boiler, melt the beeswax until it is completely smooth. Add in the remaining ingredients (except for the essential oils) one at a time, mixing them in thoroughly (you don't want there to be any lumps in the mix at all.)

After you have thoroughly blended the ingredients, add the essential oils in next, and also stir them in until the mix is completely smooth. Remove from heat and allow to cool slightly, stirring the entire time.

Once the soap has cooled enough to touch, transfer from your double boiler to a soap dispenser, and use frequently on any burns you have.

Miracle Cream
What you will need:

12 drops goldenseal oil

10 drops lemongrass oil

¼ cup aloe

1 tablespoon beeswax

1 cup unscented castile soap

1 tablespoon glycerin

¼ cup distilled water

Directions:

Using either a double boiler or a homemade double boiler, melt the beeswax until it is completely smooth. Add in the remaining ingredients (except for the essential oils) one at a time, mixing them in thoroughly (you don't want there to be any lumps in the mix at all.)

After you have thoroughly blended the ingredients, add the essential oils in next, and also stir them in until the mix is completely smooth. Remove from heat and allow to cool slightly, stirring the entire time.

Once the soap has cooled enough to touch, transfer from your double boiler to a soap dispenser, and use frequently on any burns you have.

Chapter 4 – Healing Soaps for Rashes

Rashes seem to come out of nowhere. They can be a result of an allergen, some sort of irritant, or even plants. When you have a rash of any kind, you want nothing more than to just get rid of it.

With these soaps, you are going to see your rashes disappear in no time at all, and be back to feeling like your good old self.

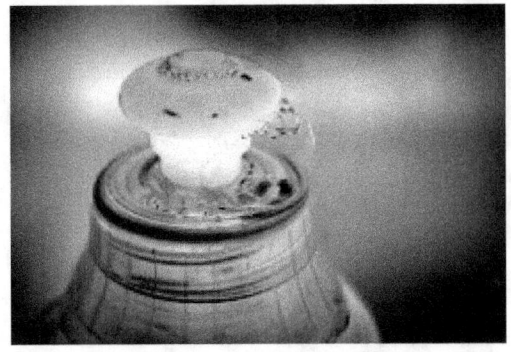

Spot Check
What you will need:

12 drops frankincense oil

10 drops myrrh oil

¼ cup aloe

1 tablespoon honey

1 tablespoon beeswax

1 cup unscented castile soap

1 tablespoon glycerin

¼ cup goat milk

Directions:

Using either a double boiler or a homemade double boiler, melt the beeswax until it is completely smooth. Add in the remaining ingredients (except for the essential oils) one at a time, mixing them in thoroughly (you don't want there to be any lumps in the mix at all.)

After you have thoroughly blended the ingredients, add the essential oils in next, and also stir them in until the mix is completely smooth. Remove from heat and allow to cool slightly, stirring the entire time.

Once the soap has cooled enough to touch, transfer from your double boiler to a soap dispenser, and use frequently on any rashes you have.

Rash Wash
What you will need:

12 drops chamomile oil

9 drops lavender oil

¼ cup aloe

1 tablespoon honey

1 tablespoon beeswax

1 cup unscented castile soap

1 tablespoon glycerin

¼ cup goat milk

Directions:

Using either a double boiler or a homemade double boiler, melt the beeswax until it is completely smooth. Add in the remaining ingredients (except for the essential oils) one at a time, mixing them in thoroughly (you don't want there to be any lumps in the mix at all.)

After you have thoroughly blended the ingredients, add the essential oils in next, and also stir them in until the mix is completely smooth. Remove from heat and allow to cool slightly, stirring the entire time.

Once the soap has cooled enough to touch, transfer from your double boiler to a soap dispenser, and use frequently on any rashes you have.

Itch It
What you will need:

12 drops peppermint oil

12 drops spearmint oil

¼ cup aloe

1 tablespoon honey

1 tablespoon beeswax

1 cup unscented castile soap

1 tablespoon glycerin

¼ cup goat milk

Directions:

Using either a double boiler or a homemade double boiler, melt the beeswax until it is completely smooth. Add in the remaining ingredients (except for the essential oils) one at a time, mixing them in thoroughly (you don't want there to be any lumps in the mix at all.)

After you have thoroughly blended the ingredients, add the essential oils in next, and also stir them in until the mix is completely smooth. Remove from heat and allow to cool slightly, stirring the entire time.

Once the soap has cooled enough to touch, transfer from your double boiler to a soap dispenser, and use frequently on any rashes you have.

Something Swell
What you will need:

10 drops geranium oil

10 drops ylang ylang oil

¼ cup aloe

1 tablespoon honey

1 tablespoon beeswax

1 cup unscented castile soap

1 tablespoon glycerin

¼ cup goat milk

Directions:

Using either a double boiler or a homemade double boiler, melt the beeswax until it is completely smooth. Add in the remaining ingredients (except for the essential oils) one at a time, mixing them in thoroughly (you don't want there to be any lumps in the mix at all.)

After you have thoroughly blended the ingredients, add the essential oils in next, and also stir them in until the mix is completely smooth. Remove from heat and allow to cool slightly, stirring the entire time.

Once the soap has cooled enough to touch, transfer from your double boiler to a soap dispenser, and use frequently on any rashes you have.

Happy Days
What you will need:

12 drops helychirsum oil

8 drops vetiver oil

¼ cup aloe

1 tablespoon honey

1 tablespoon beeswax

1 cup unscented castile soap

1 tablespoon glycerin

¼ cup goat milk

Directions:

Using either a double boiler or a homemade double boiler, melt the beeswax until it is completely smooth. Add in the remaining ingredients (except for the essential oils) one at a time, mixing them in thoroughly (you don't want there to be any lumps in the mix at all.)

After you have thoroughly blended the ingredients, add the essential oils in next, and also stir them in until the mix is completely smooth. Remove from heat and allow to cool slightly, stirring the entire time.

Once the soap has cooled enough to touch, transfer from your double boiler to a soap dispenser, and use frequently on any rashes you have.

Spring Fever

What you will need:

12 drops spearmint oil

12 drops wintergreen oil

¼ cup aloe

1 tablespoon honey

1 tablespoon beeswax

1 cup unscented castile soap

1 tablespoon glycerin

¼ cup goat milk

Directions:

Using either a double boiler or a homemade double boiler, melt the beeswax until it is completely smooth. Add in the remaining ingredients (except for the essential oils) one at a time, mixing them in thoroughly (you don't want there to be any lumps in the mix at all.)

After you have thoroughly blended the ingredients, add the essential oils in next, and also stir them in until the mix is completely smooth. Remove from heat and allow to cool slightly, stirring the entire time.

Once the soap has cooled enough to touch, transfer from your double boiler to a soap dispenser, and use frequently on any rashes you have.

Chapter 5 – Healing Soaps for Irritated Skin

Let's face it, there are times when you skin is irritated, and you just don't know why. Here are a few recipes for soothing oils that will leave your skin feeling back to its wonderful self.

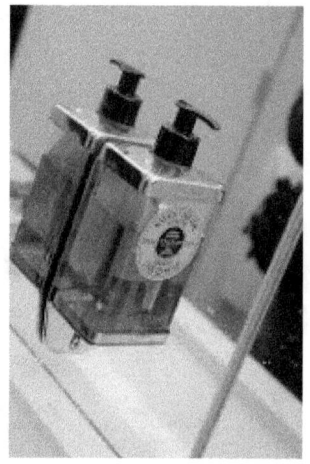

That Hits the Spot
What you will need:

12 drops eucalyptus oil

9 drops geranium oil

2 tablespoons olive oil

1 cup unscented castile soap

2 tablespoons shea butter

1 tablespoon glycerin

¼ cup distilled water

Directions:

Using either a double boiler or a homemade double boiler, melt the shea butter until it is completely smooth. Add in the remaining ingredients (except for the essential oils) one at a time, mixing them in thoroughly (you don't want there to be any lumps in the mix at all.)

After you have thoroughly blended the ingredients, add the essential oils in next, and also stir them in until the mix is completely smooth. Remove from heat and allow to cool slightly, stirring the entire time.

Once the soap has cooled enough to touch, transfer from your double boiler to a soap dispenser, and use frequently on any irritated skin you have.

Going Green
What you will need:

12 drops tea tree oil

10 drops sage oil

2 tablespoons olive oil

1 cup unscented castile soap

2 tablespoons shea butter

1 tablespoon glycerin

¼ cup distilled water

Directions:

Using either a double boiler or a homemade double boiler, melt the shea butter until it is completely smooth. Add in the remaining ingredients (except for the essential oils) one at a time, mixing them in thoroughly (you don't want there to be any lumps in the mix at all.)

After you have thoroughly blended the ingredients, add the essential oils in next, and also stir them in until the mix is completely smooth. Remove from heat and allow to cool slightly, stirring the entire time.

Once the soap has cooled enough to touch, transfer from your double boiler to a soap dispenser, and use frequently on any irritated skin you have.

The Adventurer's Tonic
What you will need:

12 drops chamomile oil

11 drops bergamot oil

2 tablespoons olive oil

1 cup unscented castile soap

2 tablespoons shea butter

1 tablespoon glycerin

¼ cup distilled water

Directions:

Using either a double boiler or a homemade double boiler, melt the shea butter until it is completely smooth. Add in the remaining ingredients (except for the essential oils) one at a time, mixing them in thoroughly (you don't want there to be any lumps in the mix at all.)

After you have thoroughly blended the ingredients, add the essential oils in next, and also stir them in until the mix is completely smooth. Remove from heat and allow to cool slightly, stirring the entire time.

Once the soap has cooled enough to touch, transfer from your double boiler to a soap dispenser, and use frequently on any irritated skin you have.

Miraculous Magic
What you will need:

8 drops neem oil

12 drops vetiver oil

2 tablespoons olive oil

1 cup unscented castile soap

2 tablespoons shea butter

1 tablespoon glycerin

¼ cup distilled water

Directions:

Using either a double boiler or a homemade double boiler, melt the shea butter until it is completely smooth. Add in the remaining ingredients (except for the essential oils) one at a time, mixing them in thoroughly (you don't want there to be any lumps in the mix at all.)

After you have thoroughly blended the ingredients, add the essential oils in next, and also stir them in until the mix is completely smooth. Remove from heat and allow to cool slightly, stirring the entire time.

Once the soap has cooled enough to touch, transfer from your double boiler to a soap dispenser, and use frequently on any irritated skin you have.

Wash It Off
What you will need:

12 drops lavender oil

8 drops rose oil

2 tablespoons olive oil

1 cup unscented castile soap

2 tablespoons shea butter

1 tablespoon glycerin

¼ cup distilled water

Directions:

Using either a double boiler or a homemade double boiler, melt the shea butter until it is completely smooth. Add in the remaining ingredients (except for the essential oils) one at a time, mixing them in thoroughly (you don't want there to be any lumps in the mix at all.)

After you have thoroughly blended the ingredients, add the essential oils in next, and also stir them in until the mix is completely smooth. Remove from heat and allow to cool slightly, stirring the entire time.

Once the soap has cooled enough to touch, transfer from your double boiler to a soap dispenser, and use frequently on any irritated skin you have.

The Soothing Slime
What you will need:

12 drops rose oil

10 drops rosewood oil

2 tablespoons olive oil

1 cup unscented castile soap

2 tablespoons shea butter

1 tablespoon glycerin

¼ cup distilled water

Directions:

Using either a double boiler or a homemade double boiler, melt the shea butter until it is completely smooth. Add in the remaining ingredients (except for the essential oils) one at a time, mixing them in thoroughly (you don't want there to be any lumps in the mix at all.)

After you have thoroughly blended the ingredients, add the essential oils in next, and also stir them in until the mix is completely smooth. Remove from heat and allow to cool slightly, stirring the entire time.

Once the soap has cooled enough to touch, transfer from your double boiler to a soap dispenser, and use frequently on any irritated skin you have.

Conclusion

There you have it, everything you need to make your own soaps and treat any kind of skin condition you may experience. I hope this book gives you the inspiration that you need to make your own soaps, no matter what your skin condition is.

This book has everything you need to take care of all your skin care ailments, and it's going to change the way you view the soap that you make. Get ready to pamper yourself in a whole new way.

Good luck, and have a happy cleaning!

FREE Bonus Reminder

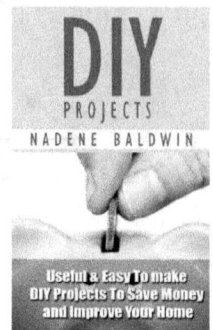

If you have not grabbed it yet, please go ahead and download your special bonus report *"DIY Projects. 13 Useful & Easy To Make DIY Projects To Save Money & Improve Your Home!"*

Simply Click the Button Below

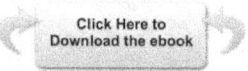

OR **Go to This Page**

http://diyhomecraft.com/free

BONUS #2: More Free & Discounted Books or Products

Do you want to receive more Free/Discounted Books or Products?

We have a mailing list where we send out our new Books or Products when they go free or with a discount on Amazon. Click on the link below to sign up for Free & Discount Book & Product Promotions.

=> Sign Up for Free & Discount Book & Product Promotions <=

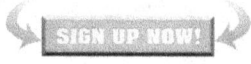

OR Go to this URL

http://zbit.ly/1WBb1Ek